401 SEXUAL ADDICTION AFFIRMATIONS: GUIDED POSITIVE MEDITATIONS FOR RE-FOCUSING YOUR SEXUAL ENERGY

A SEX ADDICTS SELF HELP MEDITATION HYPNOSIS W/ BONUS SOOTHING NATURE SOUNDS AND TONES

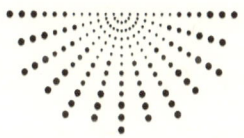

DAVID WHITEHEAD

SILK PUBLISHING

INTRODUCTION

> Just as a heroin addict chases a substance-induced high, sex addicts are bingeing on chemicals — in this case, their own hormones.
>
> — **ALEXANDRA KATEHAKIS**

Sexual addiction, also called hyper-sexuality, hyper-sexual disorder, and sexual compulsivity, is a behavioral addiction focused on sex and sexual fantasy. A sexual addiction is most often characterized by a vicious circle of hyper-sexuality and low self-esteem. Although sex can bring short-term relief, the harm to the person's psychological well-being will often increase and worsen over time.

INTRODUCTION

A person does not have to engage in extreme or "strange" sex to have an addiction. They will simply be unable to stop themselves despite the harm that they know may result from their behavior. Recovery from addictive behaviours cannot be done by anyone else. Even with a team of the best therapists in the world, you are the only person who can change yourself. With addiction, you have to want recovery and be willing to put in the time, energy and thought required to make the change.

Affirmations are short, positive messages that you repeat to yourself with the goal of implanting them deep inside your subconscious, like a little seed that eventually changes the way you think and behave. It is proven that repetitive constructive affirmations attract positive energies in your life, and that discovering your affirmation will equip you with another tool to maintain emotional and mental resilience through this transformative period.

Follow your bliss! Achieve your bliss! Become your bliss!

1
ONE DAY AT A TIME

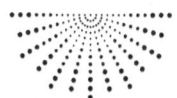

I CAN DO THIS

Affirmations work to focus your mind on the goal you want to reach, to keep you motivated and to make sure that you stay positive – to keep the image of your life without sex addiction in front of your eyes until it becomes reality.

"I CAN DO THIS."

1. I can do this.
2. I am getting stronger every day
3. I was not made to give up
4. My strength is greater than any struggle
5. I am who I want to be

6. Each day I am bettering myself
7. I discovered that I am fierce
8. I know my worth.
9. I choose what I become
10. I have decided that I am good enough
11. I've decided that I am worth it
12. I am brave enough to do this
13. No challenge is too great for me to handle
14. I have the power to change my story
15. I use failure as a stepping stone
16. I have the courage to say "no"
17. I am smart
18. I am blessed
19. I am stronger than any storm.
20. I deserve to reach my dreams
21. I am worthy of genuine love
22. I am worthy of happiness
23. Unconditional love flows through me
24. I am worthy of respect
25. I greet each day with strength
26. No matter what comes my way, I can handle it
27. I am fearless
28. I believe in myself
29. I believe in my abilities

30. Today is my day. Today I will change my life
31. I am loved
32. Unlimited energy will fill me today
33. I will be a giver of love today
34. Today, I will learn and grow
35. I will be a better person today than I was yesterday
36. Success will find me today
37. My addiction is strong, but I am stronger
38. I am grateful for another day to shine
39. I will be fearless today
40. I have done my best today
41. I am proud of myself
42. Tomorrow is a new day, filled with possibilities
43. The world is beautiful
44. I can be known for my kindness and strength
45. I am stronger than negative thoughts
46. I am not my mistakes
47. I am fully committed to achieving my goals
48. I have enough, I do enough, I am enough

49. My life is a gift, and I will use this gift with confidence and joy
50. I deserve love, compassion, and empathy
51. I choose faith over fear
52. I am creating my life exactly how I want it
53. I choose to be positive
54. I am at peace with who I am
55. I matter.
56. I act with courage and confidence
57. I live in the present, and take action to ensure a wonderful future
58. I turn my dreams into goals, and my goals into steps, and turn my steps into action
59. I am willing to change for the better
60. I allow love to fill me up and guide me in all of my actions
61. My mind is free of resistance and open to possibilities
62. I am in the process of becoming the best version of myself
63. I can do anything I put my mind to
64. I have the courage to keep going
65. I am creating the life of my dreams
66. I am totally in charge of my life

67. Whatever I put my mind to, I will achieve
68. My energy creates my reality. what I focus on, I will manifest
69. I am connected to the endless abundance of the universe
70. I make positive choices for myself
71. I love and accept myself
72. Good things happen to me all the time
73. I am productive every day.
74. I am valued.
75. Today, I will search for the good in each moment
76. I love changing, it brings me opportunity
77. I am on the path to achieving my dreams
78. I am capable
79. I am stronger than the power of any urges
80. I have the courage to do good things for myself
81. I refuse to give up on myself
82. I am purposeful
83. I was made with divine intention
84. I can, and I will
85. I feed my spirit.

86. I am in charge of how I feel today
87. I am choosing and not waiting to be chosen
88. I am enough
89. I am working on my recovery.
90. I am an imperfect yet worthwhile person.
91. I have value and worth.
92. I can love myself and accept my past.
93. I am a worthwhile person, exactly as God intended me to be.
94. I am finding my integrity one day at a time.
95. I am worthy of acceptance, exactly as I am.
96. Today, I choose to live in the moment.
97. My past actions do not define me in the present.
98. I am able to give and receive love.
99. I respect the boundaries of others.
100. I am recovering with the help of others.
101. I have done bad things, but I am not a bad person.
102. It is OK for me to talk to others about what I am thinking and feeling.
103. I am letting go of my shame.
104. I am fully present today.

105. I can heal and forgive myself for the harms I have caused.
106. I am a better person today than I was yesterday.
107. I am able to ask for and accept help when I need it, without feeling ashamed.
108. Today, I choose to reach out to others before I act out in my addiction.
109. I have compassion for myself and for others.
110. I am happy living my life one day at a time.
111. I am striving for progress, not perfection.
112. I am living a better life today than yesterday.
113. I am making positive changes in my life, one step at a time.
114. Today, my heart is clean.
115. I am fearless and rigorously honest in all aspects of life.
116. Outward failures are learning opportunities. They no longer dishearten me.
117. I am living a life of integrity.
118. Today, I am living my values.

119. Negative feelings are just feelings. They don't last.
120. I honor who I am.
121. I am worth loving. There is love all around me.
122. I am recovering and healing, one day at a time.
123. I am the right person, in the right place, at the right time.
124. Today, I choose to be myself, and to be happy with who I am.
125. I believe in myself and my abilities.
126. Today, I will do small things with great love.
127. My recovery works when I work it.
128. I am worth the effort of recovery.
129. I am responsible for the effort, not the outcome.
130. Today, I am stronger than my addiction.
131. I like myself.
132. Happiness is within me.
133. My life belongs to me, not my addiction.
134. I appreciate and cherish the true me more and more each day.
135. I am a happy, peaceful person.

136. I am a strong person with healthy habits.
137. I am capable of healthy relationships with others.
138. Today, I am walking the right path.
139. All of my problems have a solution.
140. I am proud of myself.
141. I deserve to be sober and to heal.
142. I can and I will.
143. Today, I have a choice. And the choice I make is sobriety.
144. When troubled, I can stop, breathe, and reach out for help.
145. I am full of potential
146. I add something special to this world
147. I am confident in my abilities to make a positive difference
148. I deeply and completely accept myself
149. I am proud of myself for all my big and little victories.
150. My life is full of abundance and happiness
151. I am the only thing in control of my life.
152. My life is free of addiction.
153. I can look inside myself as a source of joy.

154. I am stronger than temptation.
155. I am proud of myself.
156. I respect my body and my loved ones.
157. Every day, in every way, I am getting better.
158. I can and I will.
159. I will choose recovery.
160. I will choose to live my life .
161. I am more than capable.
162. I will show myself love,grace, and care because I deserve it.
163. I have a life and today I choose to recover and live.
164. I will be a better me.
165. I am worthy of great things.
166. I like the person I'm becoming.
167. I am loved
168. I am brave.
169. I am in touch with my emotions.
170. I deserve happiness and love.

2
AFFIRMATIONS FOR SEX ADDICTION

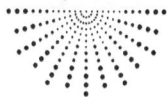

I AM FREE OF SEX ADDICTION

As a sex addict, sexual thoughts, romantic fantasies, and seductive planning can fill your mind and distort your thinking. Sex becames a way to escape your feelings and responsibilities. An important first step is to first admit you are powerless over addictive sexual behavior—that your life has become unmanageable.

You cannot let addiction win.

"I AM FREE OF SEX ADDICTION"

1. I am free from sex addiction
2. Sex addiction will no longer control my life

3. I am dedicated to overcoming my addiction to sex
4. I am always in control of my sexual urges
5. I am no longer seeing others as sex objects
6. I am living a life free from sex addiction
7. I am developing a strong will power
8. I find it easy to say NO to my own sexual urges
9. I am 100% in control of my own life
10. I have a healthy attitude towards sex
11. I forgive myself for what I have done
12. I will avoid situations that will hinder my road to recovery from sex addiction.
13. Sex addiction does not serve me.
14. I will fight my addiction.
15. I will not let sex addiction cause me to hurt my partner.
16. Recovering from addiction allows me to give back to others, which in turn helps me further my recovery.
17. I am not just a body—I am body, mind, and soul.

18. I am not a burden to others if I ask for help or support.
19. I will not worry about tomorrow as I am living for today and the present.
20. I am letting go of my addiction to sex
21. I always take responsibility for my own actions
22. I am becoming more free of sex addiction
23. I will become more in control of my sexual urges
24. I am finding myself more positive about overcoming my addiction
25. I am turning into someone who is in control of their urges
26. I am becoming someone with a strong will power
27. I deserve respect in my relationships.
28. I choose to forgive myself for the mistakes I have made, and have learned from each one.
29. I believe I can overcome sex addiction
30. I will take responsibility for my own actions
31. I am transforming into someone with a healthy attitude towards sex

32. I will see people as human beings and not as sex objects
33. I find it easy to control my sexual urges
34. I will live a life free from sex addiction
35. I will not let sex addiction intefere with my life
36. I value my loved ones; I will not let sex addiction stop me from being there for them.
37. Overcoming sex addiction is the easiest thing in the world
38. I have strong self control that allows me to overcome any habit or addiction
39. I have no need to sleep with loads of people.
40. I can fulfil myself sexually with just one partner.
41. I see the people as humans and not as sex objects
42. I will not taint all my interactions with others with sexual advances
43. I will control myself in the workplace.
44. Others see me as someone who takes responsibility for their actions
45. My life is naturally coming into balance now that I am sex addiction free.

46. The longer I remain free of addiction the happier and healthier I become.
47. I am grateful for the support I have in remaining free of sex addiction.
48. Everyone is cheering for me to remain free of sex addiction. I am grateful for the support.
49. Today and everyday I choose my health and happiness over my previous addictions.
50. I enjoy my life immensely now that I am free of sex addiction
51. I cultivate tools and treasures to support my excellent sexual health.
52. 100% of my focus is on my health and happiness. I am sex addiction free naturally
53. Being addiction free comes naturally to me.
54. I am grateful for each day that I am free of sex addiction.
55. I enjoy a sex addiction free lifestyle.
56. I am turning into someone who is in control of their life
57. I bravely strive to better myself. Addiction will not defeat me

58. My life is happy, healthy, and addiction free.
59. Every day that I am free of sex addiction, my life gets better and better.
60. I am psyched to say that I am addiction free, naturally.
61. I am proud of myself for choosing to release the things in my life that no longer serve me.
62. I am grateful that I know longer choose to participate in patterns that are harmful to my health and happiness.
63. I am committed to remaining free of addictions.
64. My life is filled with an abundance of excitement and joy
65. Today is a beautiful day to be alive and healthy.
66. I am thrilled to be addiction free naturally.
67. Life fills me with joy and pleasure.
68. I am excited to be alive at this moment.
69. I enjoy the health benefits that I receive from being free of sex addiction.
70. I value my own health and happiness and make excellent lifestyle choices.

71. I enjoy making choices that support my own health and happiness.
72. Each decision I make supports my desire to live a healthy and filling life.
73. I am delighted to be free of any and all previous addictions.
74. I love and cherish myself and therefore make life-affirming healthy choices.
75. The lifestyle choices I make are in alignment with my health and happiness.
76. I am capable of healthy relationships
77. Today, I have a choice. And the choice I make is to be free of my sex addiction
78. I deserve my freedom from sex addiction
79. My life belongs to me, not my addiction.
80. My recovery works when I work it.
81. My freedom from sex addiction is a journey, not a destination. Today I will enjoy the journey.
82. I am worth the effort of recovery.
83. I am responsible for the effort, not the outcome
84. I am recovering and healing, one day at a time.

85. Today, I choose to reach out to others before I act out on my addiction.
86. I choose peace rather than the unrest that comes with my addiction.
87. I cross the bridge of my sexual addiction and explore new possibilities of a life free of my addiction.
88. In my journey to freedom from sex addiction, in everything I do I flow and don't force.
89. I am healed and I am a healer.
90. I am part of the solution and not the problem.
91. Today I show up, grow up, give up and own up.
92. Today I am new. Today I am free of my addiction.
93. The only thing in control of my life is myself
94. I find it easy to turn down sex
95. I deserve to be free of sex addiction
96. Being surrounded by positive people is natural to me
97. My life is free from sex addiction
98. People see me as someone who has successfully overcome sex addiction
99. People look up to me as someone who

has wrestled with sex addiction and come out on top
100. Being free of sex has been an improvement in my life
101. I look inside myself for happiness
102. I am in control of my own life
103. I find it easy to turn down sex
104. I believe in my ability to recover.
105. I am not tempted at all by sex
106. I have the natural ability to stay in control
107. I always make sure to only align myself with people who support me.
108. I respect my body and my loved ones.
109. Every day, in every way, I am getting better.
110. I can look inside myself as a source of joy.
111. I am stronger than temptation,
112. I deserve great things, I will not let sex addiction deprive me of what I deserve.
113. I can and I will defeat this addiction
114. I will heal from this, I will be a better me.
115. All of my problems can be solved, I will never stop trying.
116. I am on the right path. I will keep going

117. I am in charge of my life story.
118. I will stay away from pornographic material
119. I do not need sex to feel better about myself
120. There is more to life than sexual gratification.
121. People are more than sex objects; I will be kind to them
122. I will avoid compromising sexual situations
123. I will forgive myself, my past has no hold over me.
124. I will make amends, I will right the wrongs sex addiction caused.
125. I will do right by myself and my loved ones.
126. I am happy with who I am
127. I find happiness within me
128. I am healing myself, one day at a time.
129. I am capable of getting and staying sober.
130. I am taking my life in my own hands
131. I am taking care of my body
132. I am loved by people in my life
133. I don't need sex to be happy and in peace with myself

134. I can deal with anything that comes my way
135. I am able to stay in control
136. I surround myself with people who support me
137. I am about to start a new life, free from sex addiction
138. I am becoming stronger with each passing day
139. I will take responsibility for my life
140. I will forgive myself for everything I've done
141. I appreciate and cherish myself more and more every day
142. I am becoming a strong individual with healthy habits
143. I will take control of my life. I make choices that are beneficial for me and that serve my highest good.
144. I am strong enough to recover.
145. I am proud of myself and my recovery.
146. Everyday is an opportunity to break free of sex addiction
147. I will avoid materials that will cause me to falter on my path to recovery

3
FOR YOU

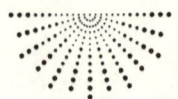

YOU MATTER

"You Matter"

1. You matter.
2. You will live a life free from sex addiction
3. You are capable of achieving anything.
4. You are getting better every day.
5. You are inspiring
6. You are worth it.
7. You are strong enough to get through this.
8. I believe in you.
9. Today is going to be a good day.
10. You are loved and appreciated.
11. You are stronger than your temptation.

12. I'm proud of you.
13. You are surrounded by people who love you.
14. You are not your mistakes.
15. Be gentle with yourself. You're doing the best you can.
16. You can do anything you put your mind to.
17. You are brave.
18. Addiction will not defeat you.
19. You have the courage to move forward.
20. You have a purpose.
21. You are in charge of what happens next.
22. I have so much faith in you.
23. I know you can overcome this.
24. No challenge is too great for you to handle.
25. I am by your side every step of the way.
26. You are worthy of happiness.
27. I love you unconditionally.
28. You deserve to succeed.
29. You are the architect of your life; You build its foundation and choose its contents
30. Today, you are brimming with energy and overflowing with joy

31. Your body is healthy; your mind is brilliant; your soul is tranquil
32. You are superior to negative thoughts and low actions
33. A river of peace washes away your addiction
34. Happiness is a choice. You base your happiness on your own accomplishments and the blessings you have been given
35. You are courageous
36. You are resilient.
37. You can change your thoughts.
38. You can fix your life.
39. Your ability to conquer your challenges is limitless
40. Your potential to succeed is infinite
41. You are courageous and you stand up for yourself
42. Your thoughts are filled with positivity and your life is plentiful with prosperity
43. Today, you abandon your old habits and take up new, more positive ones
44. You are admired
45. You are blessed with an incredible family and wonderful friends

46. You acknowledge your own self-worth; your confidence is soaring
47. You are a powerhouse; you are indestructible
48. Though these times are difficult, they are only a short phase of your life
49. Even in adversity, you shine bright as the full moon on a cloudless night.
50. You unconditionally love and accept yourself in every way.
51. You are in control of your own life
52. Today you are making peace.
53. You give yourself the freedom to speak and act honestly in every situation.
54. You have the resilience you need to achieve anything.
55. Step by step, you are releasing all fears and moving forward with your life.
56. Your life is coming together in a complete and perfect way.
57. Today you are building a life filled with possibilities more important to you than your fears.
58. Peace, abundance and self control are flowing to you right now.
59. Today you are restarting your life;

sharing your talents with a world thirsty for what you have to offer.
60. Today you are pursuing transcendent peace.
61. You have value and worth.
62. Your heart beats strong. You will win this battle
63. You have complete freedom to create your own life and you do so brilliantly each and every day.
64. Today you are giving it your all in your pursuit of recovery.
65. You are a great partner and friend. You get better and better each and every day.
66. Good things take time. You are patient and accepting in your life.
67. Good things are happening for you. Your life is moving in a positive direction.
68. You are confident in your recovery, much more confident than ever before.
69. You control your destiny.
70. You have the resilience, resourcefulness and inner strength you need to heal yourself.

71. You are undergoing a powerful, radical healing transformation.
72. Forgive yourself if today was a bad day.
73. Forgive yourself if things didn't go according to plan.
74. You are taking bold action to improve those things you want to change in your life.
75. You will gain control over your feelings and urges and you will not let them control you
76. You prioritize the habits, routines, lifestyles, and relationships that support your recovery
77. You are strong enough to prioritize your recovery
78. You are mindful
79. You can do this!
80. You will face and overcome your challenges.
81. You are living an extraordinary life.
82. You are creating peace within yourself and in your life, every day.
83. You are a model of peace and tranquility.
84. You remain, in all circumstances, calm, cool, confident, and collected.

AFTERWORD

For most people, sexual fantasies and behaviors are pathways to fun, happiness , and intimate connection. Sexual addicts, on the other hand, use these activities compulsively, and over time they lose control and have to deal with difficult life consequences as a result. Their belief systems, their self-esteem, their relationships suffer, all thanks to their addiction. If you are sexually addicted, or you think that someone you know and care about is sexually addicted, I hope that the affirmations in this book will contribute to the process of recovery, healing and reforming meaningful connections and restoring value to your life.

One day at a time.

www.ingramcontent.com/pod-product-compliance
Lightning Source LLC
Chambersburg PA
CBHW021452070526
44577CB00002B/383